The Heart of a Healer:
Daily Devotions for Christian Nurses

Contents

Introduction

As a nurse, you are often the first point of contact for patients and their families during times of illness and crisis. In these moments, you are called to provide not only physical care but also emotional and spiritual support.

The demands of this profession can be overwhelming, but as a Christian nurse, you have a unique perspective that can help you navigate these challenges. This book of 21 devotionals is designed to help you draw strength from God and deepen your faith as you care for others.

Each day, you'll find a scripture passage, a reflection on a specific aspect of nursing, and a prayer to help you connect with God and find peace in the midst of your busy schedule. These devotionals are not meant to replace your personal Bible study and prayer time, but rather to complement it and provide a daily source of encouragement.

Through this book, you will be reminded of the importance of caring for yourself, both physically and spiritually, so that you can better care for others. You'll be encouraged to seek wisdom and guidance from God as you make difficult decisions and face challenging situations. And you'll be reminded of the impact you can have on the lives of those around you as you reflect God's love and compassion in your work.

As you read these devotionals, I pray that you will find renewed strength and purpose in your work as a nurse. May God bless you as you seek to serve others with love and compassion.

Surrendering to God's Will

"Trust in the Lord with all your heart and lean not on your own understanding; in all your ways submit to him, and he will make your paths straight." - Proverbs 3:5-6 (NIV)

As a nurse, you're often faced with situations that are beyond your control. You may encounter patients with complex medical conditions or emotional needs that are difficult to address. In those moments, it's easy to feel overwhelmed and unsure of what to do. But God's Word reminds us to trust in Him and to surrender our will to His. He promises to guide us and make our paths straight.

Surrendering to God's will is not always easy. It requires us to let go of our own plans and desires and to trust that God knows what's best for us. But when we do surrender to Him, we find peace and rest in His loving arms. We can trust that He will never leave us or forsake us and that He is always working for our good.

As you begin your workday, take a moment to surrender your plans and your patients to God. Ask Him to guide you and give you wisdom as you care for those in need. Remember that you are not alone and that God is with you every step of the way.

Prayer:

Heavenly Father, I come before you today and surrender my will to yours. I trust that you know what is best for me and for my patients. Help me to lean on you and to trust in your guidance and wisdom. Give me the strength to face the challenges of the day and the compassion to care for those in need. Thank you for your love and grace, and for the privilege of serving as a nurse.

In Jesus' name, amen.

Extending Grace to Others

"Therefore, as God's chosen people, holy and dearly loved, clothe yourselves with compassion, kindness, humility, gentleness, and patience." - Colossians 3:12 (NIV)

As a nurse, you have the opportunity to show compassion and extend grace to those around you. Your patients may be in pain, afraid, or feeling vulnerable, and your kind words and actions can make a big difference in their experience. But extending grace isn't always easy, especially when you are dealing with difficult patients or coworkers.

God's Word reminds us that we are chosen by Him and dearly loved. He calls us to clothe ourselves with compassion, kindness, humility, gentleness, and patience. These qualities are essential for showing grace to others, even in the midst of challenging situations.

When we extend grace to others, we reflect the love of Christ and show His light to the world. We become agents of healing and hope, bringing comfort and peace to those who are hurting. And in doing so, we also receive grace from God, who promises to bless those who show mercy and kindness to others.

As you go about your day, ask God to help you clothe yourself with compassion, kindness, humility, gentleness, and patience. Look for opportunities to extend grace to your patients and coworkers, even when it's difficult. And remember that you are chosen and loved by God, who gives you the strength and grace to love others as He loves you.

Prayer:

Dear God, thank you for choosing me and loving me. Help me to clothe myself with compassion, kindness, humility, gentleness, and patience, and to extend grace to those around me. Give me the strength and wisdom to show your love to my patients and coworkers, even in challenging situations. And may my actions and words bring healing and hope to those who are hurting. In Jesus' name, amen.

Finding Rest in God's Presence

"Come to me, all you who are weary and burdened, and I will give you rest. Take my yoke upon you and learn from me, for I am gentle and humble in heart, and you will find rest for your souls." - Matthew 11:28-29 (NIV)

As a nurse, you can often find yourself feeling weary and burdened by the demands of your work. You may be dealing with long hours, difficult patients, and challenging situations that leave you feeling exhausted and overwhelmed. But in the midst of all of this, Jesus invites you to come to Him and find rest in His presence.

Jesus promises to give us rest when we come to Him with our burdens. He invites us to take His yoke upon us and to learn from Him, for He is gentle and humble in heart. When we take on His yoke, we discover that it is light and easy to bear. We also discover that it leads us to a beautiful place of rest and peace.

Finding rest in God's presence doesn't mean that our work as nurses will be easy or that we won't face challenges. But it does mean that we can trust in God's strength and guidance to help us through difficult times. We can find comfort and peace in knowing that God is with us and that He is working all things for our good.

As you go about your day, take a moment to come to Jesus and find rest in His presence. Ask Him to help you take on His yoke and to learn from Him so that you can find rest for your soul. And remember that no matter what challenges you may face, you can trust in God's strength and guidance to see you through.

Prayer:

Heavenly Father, I come to you today and lay my burdens at your feet. I thank you for inviting me to find rest in your presence and for promising to give me rest when I am weary and burdened. Help me to take on your yoke and to learn from you, so that I can find rest for my soul. Give me the strength and guidance I need to face the challenges of the day, and may your peace fill my heart and mind. In Jesus' name, amen.

Trusting in God's Plan

"For I know the plans I have for you," declares the Lord, "plans to prosper you and not to harm you, plans to give you hope and a future." - Jeremiah 29:11 (NIV)

As a nurse, you may encounter situations that leave you feeling uncertain and unsure of what the future holds. You may also be facing difficult decisions or struggling to find your place in your career. But in the midst of all of this, God reminds us that He has a plan for our lives.

Jeremiah 29:11 reminds us that God's plans for us are good and that He has a future filled with hope for us. Even when we may not understand what is happening in our lives, we can trust that God is in control and that He is working all things for our good.

Trusting in God's plan means letting go of our own desires and expectations, and surrendering our lives to His will. It means seeking His guidance and direction, and trusting that He will lead us down the path He has set for us. When we trust in God's plan, we find peace and security in knowing that He is with us every step of the way.

As you go about your day, take a moment to reflect on God's plan for your life. Trust in His goodness and His faithfulness, and seek His guidance as you make decisions and navigate your career as a nurse. And remember that no matter what challenges you may face, God has a plan for your life that is filled with hope and a future.

Prayer:

Dear God, I thank you for the plans you have for my life. Help me to trust in your goodness and your faithfulness, and to seek your guidance as I make decisions and navigate my career as a nurse. Give me peace and security in knowing that you are with me every step of the way and that you are working all things for my good. In Jesus' name, amen.

Serving with Humility

"Do nothing out of selfish ambition or vain conceit. Rather, in humility value others above yourselves, not looking to your own interests but each of you to the interests of the others." - Philippians 2:3-4 (NIV)

As a nurse, you are called to serve others with compassion and care. But sometimes, it can be easy to fall into the trap of serving out of selfish ambition or seeking recognition for your work. However, God's Word reminds us to serve with humility and to value others above ourselves.

Jesus himself modeled humility and servanthood throughout His life on earth. He washed the feet of His disciples, healed the sick, and served those around Him with compassion and love. He calls us to follow His example, to look to the interests of others, and to serve with a heart of humility.

Serving with humility means putting the needs of others before our own desires for recognition or success. It means recognizing the value and worth of every person we encounter, and treating them with dignity and respect. When we serve with humility, we reflect the love of Christ to those around us and bring glory to His name.

As you go about your day, ask God to help you serve with humility and to value others above yourself. Look for opportunities to serve those around you with compassion and care, and remember that your work as a nurse is a reflection of your faith in Christ.

Prayer:

Dear God, thank you for the opportunity to serve others as a nurse. Help me to serve with humility and to value others above myself. Teach me to look to the interests of others and to treat them with compassion and care. May my work bring glory to your name and reflect the love of Christ to those around me. In Jesus' name, amen.

Finding Strength in God's Word

"All Scripture is God-breathed and is useful for teaching, rebuking, correcting and training in righteousness, so that the servant of God may be thoroughly equipped for every good work." - 2 Timothy 3:16-17 (NIV)

As a nurse, you may face long hours, difficult patients, and challenging situations. But in the midst of all of this, God's Word provides us with strength and encouragement. 2 Timothy 3:16-17 reminds us that all Scripture is God-breathed and useful for teaching, rebuking, correcting, and training in righteousness.

God's Word is a source of comfort and guidance, and it equips us to do every good work. When we spend time in His Word, we are strengthened and renewed, and we are better able to serve those around us with compassion and care.

Finding strength in God's Word means making time to read and meditate on His Word. It means seeking His wisdom and guidance and allowing His truth to transform our hearts and minds. When we allow God's Word to shape our thoughts and actions, we are better equipped to face the challenges of our day-to-day lives.

As you go about your day, take a moment to reflect on the power of God's Word in your life. Make time to read and meditate on His Word, and allow His truth to transform your heart and mind. And remember that in His Word, you will find strength and encouragement to face whatever challenges may come your way.

Prayer:

Dear God, thank you for the power of your Word in my life. Help me to make time to read and meditate on your Word, and to seek your wisdom and guidance in all that I do. May your truth transform my heart and mind, and equip me to do every good work. In Jesus' name, amen.

Practicing Gratitude

"Give thanks in all circumstances; for this is God's will for you in Christ Jesus." - 1 Thessalonians 5:18 (NIV)

As a nurse, you may encounter challenging situations that can leave you feeling stressed or overwhelmed. But even in the midst of difficult circumstances, we can find joy and peace by practicing gratitude.

1 Thessalonians 5:18 reminds us to give thanks in all circumstances, for this is God's will for us in Christ Jesus. When we practice gratitude, we shift our focus away from our problems and onto the blessings in our lives. We begin to see the good in every situation, and we find joy and contentment in even the smallest things.

Practicing gratitude means intentionally looking for things to be thankful for, even in difficult circumstances. It means focusing on the positive instead of the negative and choosing to see the good in every situation. When we practice gratitude, we cultivate a heart of thanksgiving, and we begin to see God's goodness and faithfulness in all areas of our lives.

As you go about your day, take a moment to reflect on the blessings in your life. Practice gratitude by thanking God for even the smallest things, and by focusing on the positive instead of the negative. And remember that when we practice gratitude, we find joy and contentment, and we cultivate a heart of thanksgiving that honors and glorifies God.

Prayer:

Dear God, thank you for the blessings in my life. Help me to practice gratitude by focusing on the positive instead of the negative, and by thanking you for even the smallest things. May my heart be filled with thanksgiving, and may my gratitude honor and glorify you. In Jesus' name, amen.

Trusting in God's Provision

And my God will meet all your needs according to the riches of his glory in Christ Jesus." - Philippians 4:19 (NIV)

As a nurse, you may face financial challenges, work-related stress, or personal struggles that can leave you feeling anxious or overwhelmed. But in the midst of all of this, we can find peace and security by trusting in God's provision.

Philippians 4:19 reminds us that God will meet all our needs according to the riches of his glory in Christ Jesus. When we trust in God's provision, we can have confidence that he will provide for us in all areas of our lives, including our physical, emotional, and spiritual needs.

Trusting in God's provision means surrendering our worries and fears to him and placing our trust in His faithfulness. It means recognizing that God is the source of all provision and that He will provide for us in ways that are beyond our understanding.

As you go about your day, take a moment to reflect on God's provision in your life. Trust in His faithfulness, and surrender your worries and fears to Him. And remember that when we trust in God's provision, we find peace and security that comes from knowing that He is in control.

Prayer:

Dear God, thank you for your provision in my life. Help me to trust in your faithfulness, and to surrender my worries and fears to you. May I find peace and security in knowing that you are in control and that you will provide for all my needs according to the riches of your glory in Christ Jesus. In Jesus' name, amen.

Honoring God in Your Work

"Whatever you do, work at it with all your heart, as working for the Lord, not for human masters." - Colossians 3:23 (NIV)

As a nurse, you have the opportunity to make a difference in the lives of your patients and their families every day. But even in the midst of busy schedules and demanding workloads, we can honor God in our work by approaching our work as if we were working for the Lord.

Colossians 3:23 reminds us to work at everything we do with all our heart, as working for the Lord and not for human masters. When we approach our work in this way, we honor God with our attitudes and actions, and we demonstrate our commitment to serving Him in all areas of our lives.

Honoring God in our work means doing our best, even when no one is watching. It means treating our patients and colleagues with kindness and respect and demonstrating the love of Christ in all that we do. And it means recognizing that our work is not just a job, but a calling from God to serve others and make a difference in the world.

As you go about your work today, ask God to help you approach your work with the same dedication and commitment as if you were working for Him. Honor Him with your attitudes and actions, and seek to serve others with the love of Christ.

Prayer:

Dear God, thank you for the opportunity to serve others through my work as a nurse. Help me to approach my work as if I were working for you, and to honor you with my attitudes and actions. May I demonstrate the love of Christ to my patients and colleagues, and seek to make a difference in the world through the work that I do. In Jesus' name, amen.

The Heart of a Nurse

"The King will reply, 'Truly I tell you, whatever you did for one of the least of these brothers and sisters of mine, you did for me.'" - Matthew 25:40 (NIV)

As a nurse, you have the opportunity to care for the sick, the injured, and the vulnerable. You have the ability to comfort those in pain, offer hope to those who are afraid, and bring healing to those who are suffering. In doing so, you demonstrate the heart of a nurse and the heart of Christ.

In Matthew 25:40, Jesus tells us that whatever we do for the least of His brothers and sisters, we do for Him. When we care for the sick and the vulnerable, we are serving Christ Himself. And when we approach our work with compassion, kindness, and humility, we demonstrate the heart of Christ to those around us.

The heart of a nurse is a heart of service. It is a heart that seeks to put the needs of others before our own and to offer comfort and healing to those who are hurting. It is a heart that is willing to go the extra mile, to listen, to care, and to love.

As you go about your work today, ask God to help you demonstrate the heart of a nurse to those around you. May you serve others with compassion, kindness, and humility, and may you bring the love of Christ to those who are in need.

Prayer:

Dear God, thank you for the opportunity to care for the sick, the injured, and the vulnerable. Help me to demonstrate the heart of a nurse, and the heart of Christ, to those around me. May I serve others with compassion, kindness, and humility, and may I bring your love to those who are in need. In Jesus' name, amen.

Caring for the Whole Person

"What good is it, my brothers and sisters, if someone claims to have faith but has no deeds? Can such faith save them? Suppose a brother or a sister is without clothes and daily food. If one of you says to them, 'Go in peace; keep warm and well fed,' but does nothing about their physical needs, what good is it? In the same way, faith by itself, if it is not accompanied by action, is dead." - James 2:14-17 (NIV)

As a nurse, you have the opportunity to care for the whole person - body, mind, and spirit. You have the ability to address physical needs, offer emotional support, and provide spiritual care. In doing so, you demonstrate the love of Christ and the importance of caring for the whole person.

In James 2:14-17, we are reminded that faith without deeds is dead. It is not enough to simply say that we care for the sick and the vulnerable; we must also take action to meet their physical, emotional, and spiritual needs. As nurses, we are called to care for the whole person, and to offer holistic care that addresses all aspects of their well-being.

Caring for the whole person means taking the time to listen, understand, and provide personalized care that meets their unique needs. It means addressing physical symptoms, offering emotional support, and providing spiritual care when appropriate. It also means recognizing that each person is made in the image of God and deserves to be treated with dignity and respect.

As you go about your work today, ask God to help you care for the whole person. May you take the time to listen, understand, and provide personalized care to each of them. And may you demonstrate the love of Christ to those around you.

Prayer:

Dear God, I thank you for the opportunity to care for the whole person as a nurse. Help me to listen, understand, and provide personalized care that meets the unique needs of each person I encounter. May I offer holistic care that addresses all aspects of their well-being, and may I demonstrate the love of Christ to those around me. In Jesus' name, amen.

Loving Like Jesus

"A new command I give you: Love one another. As I have loved you, so you must love one another. By this everyone will know that you are my disciples if you love one another." - John 13:34-35 (NIV)

As a nurse, you have the opportunity to love like Jesus every day. You can offer compassion, kindness, and selflessness to those in your care, and demonstrate the love of Christ in all that you do. In John 13:34-35, Jesus commands us to love one another, just as He has loved us. And by doing so, we demonstrate to the world that we are His disciples.

Loving like Jesus means putting the needs of others before our own, and showing genuine care and concern for their well-being. It means treating each person with respect and dignity, regardless of their background or circumstances. It also means offering grace and forgiveness when others fall short, just as Christ has done for us.

As you go about your work today, ask God to help you love like Jesus. May you offer compassion, kindness, and selflessness to those in your care, and demonstrate the love of Christ in all that you do. May others see your love and recognize that you are a disciple of Jesus.

Prayer:

Dear God, thank you for the example of Jesus, who loved us and gave himself up for us. Help me to love like Jesus in all that I do, putting the needs of others before my own and showing genuine care and concern for their well-being. May I treat each person with respect and dignity, and offer grace and forgiveness when others fall short. And may others see my love and recognize that I am a disciple of Jesus. In Jesus' name, amen.

Running the Race with Perseverance

"Therefore, since we are surrounded by such a great cloud of witnesses, let us throw off everything that hinders and the sin that so easily entangles. And let us run with perseverance the race marked out for us, fixing our eyes on Jesus, the pioneer, and perfecter of faith." - Hebrews 12:1-2 (NIV)

Nursing can be a demanding and challenging profession, requiring physical, emotional, and mental strength. But as Christian nurses, we can find strength in God as we run the race of life with perseverance. In Hebrews 12:1-2, we are reminded to throw off everything that hinders us, including sin, and to fix our eyes on Jesus, the pioneer, and perfecter of our faith.

Running the race of life with perseverance means persevering in the face of challenges and obstacles, and continuing to trust in God's strength and guidance. It means putting aside distractions and sins that can hinder our progress, and focusing on the path that God has marked out for us. It also means keeping our eyes fixed on Jesus, who ran the race before us and endured the cross for the joy set before Him.

As you go about your work today, remember to run the race with perseverance. Throw off everything that hinders you, and fix your eyes on Jesus. May you find strength and endurance in Him, and trust that He will guide you through every challenge and obstacle you may face.

Prayer:

Dear God, thank you for the strength and guidance you offer us as we run the race of life. Help me to throw off everything that hinders me, and to fix my eyes on Jesus, the pioneer, and perfecter of my faith. Give me the perseverance I need to trust in your strength and guidance and to keep running the race even in the face of challenges and obstacles. In Jesus' name, amen.

Overcoming Challenges with Faith

"No, in all these things we are more than conquerors through him who loved us. For I am convinced that neither death nor life, neither angels nor demons, neither the present nor the future, nor any powers, neither height nor depth, nor anything else in all creation, will be able to separate us from the love of God that is in Christ Jesus our Lord." - Romans 8:37-39 (NIV)

As a nurse, you may face many challenges and obstacles in your work. But as a Christian nurse, you have the assurance that nothing can separate you from the love of God. In Romans 8:37-39, we are reminded that we are more than conquerors through Christ and that nothing in all creation can separate us from His love.

Overcoming challenges with faith means trusting in God's love and provision, even in the face of difficult circumstances. It means recognizing that we are not alone in our struggles and that God is with us every step of the way. It also means holding onto the hope and assurance that nothing can separate us from the love of God that is in Christ Jesus.

As you go about your work today, remember to overcome challenges with faith. Trust in God's love and provision, and hold onto the hope and assurance that nothing can separate you from Him. May you find strength and peace in his presence, and may you be a source of hope and encouragement to those in your care.

Prayer:

Dear God, thank you for the assurance that nothing can separate me from your love. Help me to overcome challenges with faith, trusting in your provision, and holding onto the hope and assurance that comes from knowing you. May I find strength and peace in your presence, and be a source of hope and encouragement to those in my care. In Jesus' name, amen.

Finding Strength in God's Grace

"But he said to me, 'My grace is sufficient for you, for my power is made perfect in weakness.' Therefore, I will boast all the more gladly about my weaknesses, so that Christ's power may rest on me. That is why, for Christ's sake, I delight in weaknesses, in insults, in hardships, in persecutions, in difficulties. For when I am weak, then I am strong." - 2 Corinthians 12:9-10 (NIV)

As a nurse, you may feel like you need to have it all together, to always be strong and capable for your patients. But the truth is, we all have weaknesses and limitations. In 2 Corinthians 12:9-10, we are reminded that it is in our weakness that God's grace and power is made perfect.

When we recognize our weaknesses and limitations, we open ourselves up to receive God's grace and strength. It is through our struggles and difficulties that we can experience the power of Christ at work in our lives. Instead of trying to hide our weaknesses, we can boast about them, knowing that God's grace is sufficient for us.

As you go about your work today, remember to find strength in God's grace. Recognize your weaknesses and limitations, and trust in God's power to work through them. May you experience the fullness of His grace and strength in your life, and may you be a source of hope and encouragement to those in your care.

Prayer:

Dear God, thank you for your grace and strength in my life. Help me to recognize my weaknesses and limitations, and to trust in your power to work through them. May I find strength in your grace, and be a source of hope and encouragement to those in my care. In Jesus' name, amen.

Finding Joy in the Midst of Stress

"Do not be anxious about anything, but in every situation, by prayer and petition, with thanksgiving, present your requests to God. And the peace of God, which transcends all understanding, will guard your hearts and your minds in Christ Jesus." - Philippians 4:6-7 (NIV)

As a nurse, you face a lot of stress and pressure on a daily basis. It's easy to become anxious and overwhelmed with the demands of your job. But in Philippians 4:6-7, we are reminded that we don't have to be anxious about anything. We can bring all our worries and concerns to God in prayer and trust that He will give us His peace.

When we focus on our problems, we can easily become consumed by them. But when we shift our focus to God and give Him our burdens, we open ourselves up to experience His peace and joy, the type that surpasses all understanding. By taking time to pray and give thanks to God, we can find joy even in the midst of stress and difficulty.

So as you go about your work today, take time to bring your worries and concerns to God in prayer. Ask Him for His peace and strength to carry you through the day. And remember to give thanks for all the good things in your life, even amidst the challenges.

Prayer:

Dear God, thank you for your peace and joy in my life. Help me to trust in you and bring all my worries and concerns to you in prayer. May your peace guard my heart and mind in Christ Jesus, and may I find joy even in the midst of stress and difficulty. In Jesus' name, amen.

Renewing Your Mind in God's Word

"Do not conform to the pattern of this world, but be transformed by the renewing of your mind. Then you will be able to test and approve what God's will is—his good, pleasing and perfect will." - Romans 12:2 (NIV)

As a nurse, you encounter many situations that can challenge your faith and test your beliefs. It's important to renew your mind daily in God's word to stay grounded in your faith and be able to discern God's will for your life.

In Romans 12:2, we are encouraged to not conform to the pattern of this world, but to be transformed by the renewing of our minds. This means intentionally seeking out God's truth and wisdom through reading and studying the Bible, prayer, and fellowship with other believers.

By immersing yourself in God's word, you can gain a new perspective on the challenges you face as a nurse. You can find hope and encouragement in the promises of God and be reminded of His love and faithfulness. As you align your thoughts and beliefs with God's truth, you will be better equipped to discern His will for your life and make decisions that honor Him.

So today, take time to renew your mind in God's word. Read a passage of Scripture, meditate on its meaning, and ask God to speak to you through his word. Let His truth guide your thoughts and actions, and trust that He will lead you on the path of righteousness.

Prayer:

Dear God, thank you for your word that is a lamp to my feet and a light to my path. Help me to renew my mind in your truth and wisdom each day. May your word guide my thoughts and actions, and may I discern your will for my life. In Jesus' name, amen.

Being a Light in the Workplace

"You are the light of the world. A town built on a hill cannot be hidden. Neither do people light a lamp and put it under a bowl. Instead, they put it on its stand, and it gives light to everyone in the house. In the same way, let your light shine before others, that they may see your good deeds and glorify your Father in heaven."
- Matthew 5:14-16 (NIV)

As a nurse, you have the opportunity to be a light in the workplace by shining the love of Christ on those around you. Your coworkers and patients may be going through difficult times, and your positive attitude and compassionate care can make a significant impact.

In Matthew 5:14-16, Jesus calls us to be the light of the world. Just as a city on a hill cannot be hidden, our light should shine before others so that they may see our good deeds and glorify God. This means living out our faith in tangible ways, showing love and kindness to those around us, and being a positive influence in our workplace.

When you approach your work with a servant's heart and a desire to show Christ's love to others, you can make a lasting impact on those around you. Your actions and words can reflect the hope and peace that comes from a relationship with Jesus, and you can be a source of encouragement to those who are struggling.

So today, ask God to show you how to be a light in your workplace. Look for opportunities to show kindness, offer a listening ear, and speak words of encouragement to those around you. Let your light shine brightly, so that others may see your good deeds and glorify your Father in heaven.

Prayer:

Dear God, help me to be a light in my workplace, shining the love of Christ to those around me. May my actions and words reflect your hope and peace, and may I be a source of encouragement to those who are struggling. Show me how I can serve others and make a positive impact in my workplace. In Jesus' name, amen.

Sharing Your Faith with Patients

"But in your hearts revere Christ as Lord. Always be prepared to give an answer to everyone who asks you to give the reason for the hope that you have. But do this with gentleness and respect." - 1 Peter 3:15 (NIV)

As a Christian nurse, you have the unique opportunity to share your faith with your patients. Many patients are facing difficult times and may be searching for hope and meaning in their lives. By sharing the love of Christ with them, you can offer them a source of hope and peace.

In 1 Peter 3:15, we are encouraged to always be prepared to give an answer to everyone who asks us about the hope that we have. This means being intentional about sharing our faith and being prepared to give a reason for the hope that we have in Christ.

When sharing your faith with patients, it is important to do so with gentleness and respect. This means listening to their concerns and questions, sharing your own experiences in a non-judgmental way, and being respectful of their beliefs.

Remember that sharing your faith with patients is not about trying to convert them or force your beliefs on them. Instead, it is about offering them the hope and peace that comes from a relationship with Christ and being a source of comfort and encouragement in their time of need.

So today, ask God to give you the courage and wisdom to share your faith with your patients. Look for opportunities to offer them words of encouragement and share your own experiences of God's love and faithfulness. And remember to do so with gentleness and respect, always pointing them toward the hope that comes from a relationship with Christ.

Prayer:

Dear God, give me the courage and wisdom to share my faith with my patients. Help me to be a source of hope and comfort to those who are struggling, and to always point them toward the hope that comes from a relationship with Christ. Give me the words to say and the sensitivity to listen to their concerns and questions. In Jesus' name, amen.

Praying for Your Patients and Co-workers

"I urge, then, first of all, that petitions, prayers, intercession, and thanksgiving be made for all people – for kings and all those in authority, that we may live peaceful and quiet lives in all godliness and holiness. This is good, and pleases God our Savior, who wants all people to be saved and to come to a knowledge of the truth." - 1 Timothy 2:1-4 (NIV)

As a Christian nurse, you have a unique opportunity to pray for your patients and co-workers. Prayer is a powerful tool that can bring comfort, peace, and healing to those who are hurting or struggling.

In 1 Timothy 2:1-4, we are urged to pray for all people, including those in positions of authority. This includes our patients, their families, our colleagues, and those in leadership positions within our workplace. By praying for them, we are not only seeking their physical healing and well-being but also their spiritual well-being.

As you go about your work as a nurse, take time to lift up your patients and co-workers in prayer. Pray for their physical healing, emotional strength, and spiritual growth. Ask God to give them comfort, peace, and hope in their time of need. Also pray for your workplace as a whole, that it may be a place of healing, compassion, and grace.

Remember that prayer is not just a one-time thing but a continual act of faith. Make it a habit to pray for your patients and co-workers regularly, both during your workday and in your personal time.

Prayer:

Dear God, thank you for the opportunity to serve as a nurse and to care for those who are hurting and in need. Help me to remember the power of prayer and to lift up my patients and co-workers to you regularly. I pray for their physical healing, emotional strength, and spiritual growth. I ask that you would give them comfort, peace, and hope in their time of need. And I pray for my workplace, that it may be a place of healing, compassion, and grace. In Jesus' name, amen.

Seeking Wisdom from God

"If any of you lacks wisdom, you should ask God, who gives generously to all without finding fault, and it will be given to you." - James 1:5 (NIV)

As a nurse, you are faced with many difficult decisions each day. Whether it's determining the best course of treatment for a patient or navigating complex ethical issues, you need wisdom to make the right choices. Fortunately, James 1:5 reminds us that we can ask God for wisdom, and He will give it generously.

God is the source of all wisdom, and He desires to give us the guidance we need to make wise decisions. But we must be willing to seek His wisdom and trust that He will provide it. This requires humility and a willingness to surrender our own understanding and ideas to God's will.

So, when you find yourself facing a difficult decision, take time to seek God's wisdom. Ask Him for guidance and clarity, and trust that He will provide it in His perfect timing. Also, remember that wisdom is not just about making the right decision, but also about living in a way that honors God and reflects His love to those around us.

Prayer:

Dear God, thank you for the gift of wisdom and for your promise to give it generously when we ask. Help me to seek your wisdom in every decision I make as a nurse, and to trust that you will guide me in the right direction. Give me humility and a willingness to surrender my own understanding to your will. And help me to live in a way that honors you and reflects your love to those around me. In Jesus' name, amen.

Conclusion

Remember, being a Christian nurse is both a calling and a privilege. The demands of this profession can be daunting, but with God's help, you can rise to the challenge and make a meaningful difference in the lives of those you serve. This book of devotionals has been written to encourage and equip you as you seek to live out your faith in the workplace.

Through these devotionals, we have explored various aspects of nursing, from caring for the whole person to sharing your faith with patients. We have been reminded of the importance of seeking God's wisdom, finding strength in His grace, and trusting in His provision. We have also been challenged to love like Jesus, persevere in difficult times, and be a light in the workplace.

As you continue your journey as a Christian nurse, I encourage you to seek God's guidance and strength. Let His love and compassion flow through you as you care for those in need. Remember that your work is a reflection of your faith and that every patient you care for is an opportunity to share the love of Christ.

May these devotionals inspire and equip you to serve with excellence and to bring glory to God in your work. Thank you for your dedication and service to this noble profession.

Delightful Devotionals